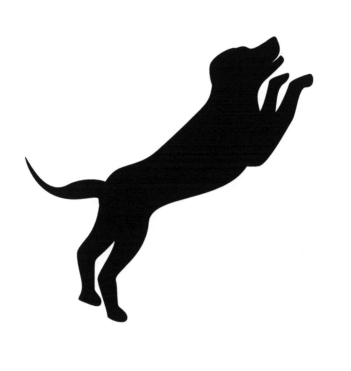

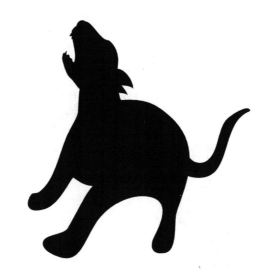

Barking Up the Right Tree

A Time-Saving Guide for Landing Your
First or Next Job as a Veterinary Nurse/Technician

Patricia M. Lee, MA

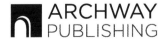
ARCHWAY
PUBLISHING

This book is a work of non-fiction. Unless otherwise noted, the author and the publisher make no explicit guarantees as to the accuracy of the information contained in this book and in some cases, names of people and places have been altered to protect their privacy.

Archway Publishing books may be ordered through booksellers or by contacting:

Archway Publishing
1663 Liberty Drive
Bloomington, IN 47403
www.archwaypublishing.com
1 (888) 242-5904

Because of the dynamic nature of the Internet, any web addresses or links contained in this book may have changed since publication and may no longer be valid. The views expressed in this work are solely those of the author and do not necessarily reflect the views of the publisher, and the publisher hereby disclaims any responsibility for them.

Any people depicted in stock imagery provided by Getty Images are models, and such images are being used for illustrative purposes only. Certain stock imagery © Getty Images.

ISBN: 978-1-4808-7486-2 (sc)
ISBN: 978-1-4808-7495-4 (e)

Library of Congress Control Number: 2019901572

Print information available on the last page.

Archway Publishing rev. date: 4/3/2019

CONTENTS

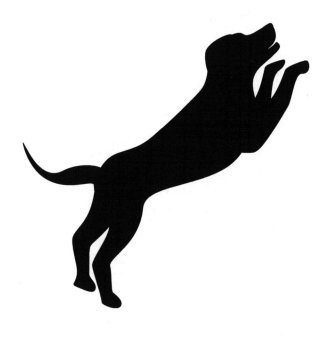

Introduction

Barking up the Right Tree is a straightforward, simple approach to securing a job in the veterinary care industry.

This book will help you focus on what's really important when it comes to finding the job of your dreams by eliminating steps that waste your time and the employer's. It will also clarify what you need to have ready prior to job searching and what you need to be prepared for a job interview at a moment's notice. No last-minute, frantic phone calls to possible references or begging for letters of recommendation or reference. You will see how having all of this at your fingertips will lessen your stress and put you in the position to be hired.

Learn how many "truths" that you believed in about resumes, job searches, and job interviews are just not getting you the job that you want in today's veterinary field job market. This book will help you avoid "barking up the wrong tree" and wasting valuable time and effort in your externship and job search activities.

You will learn the tools you will need to take with you on the interview, what to say, and more importantly, what *not* to say on an interview in the veterinary field.

Individuals who are just beginning their professional careers as well as career changers into the veterinary care field will benefit by reading this book!

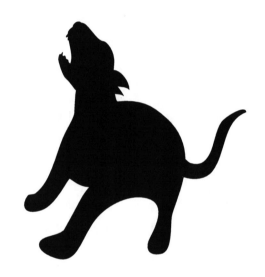

Veterinary Care Support Staff— the Backbone of Any Practice

Of course everyone knows that veterinarians are the ones you go to when you are concerned about the health of your pet. The veterinary care support staff, who are sometimes overlooked, are also veterinary professionals, and form the backbone of clinic staff. They are called by a variety of names in the veterinary field: veterinary nurses, veterinary technicians, veterinary assistants, vet tech assistants, kennel techs, research lab techs, and pre-clinical technicians, to name a few.

These professionals in the veterinary care industry allow the veterinarian to concentrate of diagnosis, prescribing drugs, and surgery. They can give injections, read blood tests, take x-rays, assist in surgery, clean teeth, anesthetize patients, and give post-operative care. But their skills don't stop there. The veterinary care support staff is also trained to answer phones, make appointments, clean cages, and provide loving care for patients in the hospital.

Much is expected of the veterinary support staff, although recognizing their importance is long overdue. Much progress has been made in veterinary field in acknowledging and utilizing these educated, well-trained professionals more than ever.

The veterinary care support staff in the veterinary industry has to be part nurse, medical technologist, radiology technician, dental hygienist, pharmacist, anesthetist, EKG technician, surgery technician, record keeper, computer, operator, inventory specialist, and several different types of counselors. The part that all of these veterinary professionals have, which can't be taught, is selfless love of animals!

Tools for the Job Search and Interview

1. The job application should be properly filled out and mistake free, online or on paper.*

2. Your resume should be mistake free, one page, concise, and organized.

3. You should have two to four references with contact information. You must first get permission from the people you want to use as references.

4. Include a letter of recommendation/reference.

5. Have a portfolio, when indicated.

6. Preparation for the interview:

    • Research the clinic/hospital.

    • Look up directions to the clinic/hospital.

    • Learn the name of the person who is interviewing you.

    • Review some sample interview questions.

7. Have an appropriate interview outfit ready to wear!

8. Have enthusiasm for the veterinary field and for the interview process.

9. Prepare a thank-you note/letter and stamps. Email thank-you's are acceptable, although a plain, professional-looking thank you card or letter, ready to send on the same day of the interview, is recommended.

10. Have an overall positive attitude.

11. Be willing to learn.

12. Your veterinary care skills and abilities are a given due to your education, although you are not expected to know everything when you first start out in the field!

Sample Job Application for Veterinary Care Position

Date:_____

Full Name: _____Previous or Maiden Name:_____

(If your name changed anytime throughout your schooling or the past ten years of employment, add your previous name.)

Address:_____

Phone(s):_____

Position applied for:_____

Availability: _____Full-time only _____ Part-time only _____ Part-time or Full-time, as needed

(Depending on the time of year, many veterinary care positions start out part-time and go into full-time. You may want to put either to get your foot in the door!)

Days and hours available to work: _____ (State you are available when needed for your best chance of getting an interview and being hired. Evenings and weekends are usually required for new hires.)

What rate of pay do you expect?_____(Attempt to find out what the position pays first, but always give a range, like twelve to fifteen dollars an hour, or put negotiable.)

What are you goals for the next two years?
_____
_____

(Employers don't really want to know about your goals and dreams. They want to know if they train you will you stay with them or move on to another position with those two years. State that your plans are to work at your position diligently and improve your skills, and become certified when indicated.)

Why do you want to work with animals?_____
_____

(Do not say, "Because I love animals!" This is obvious. Briefly state your reason for assisting animals through your education and training, and state something specific about the facility.)

Most Recent School You attended:_____

Degree or Certificate Received:_____year_____

Do you have any special skills or awards, or relevant experiences we should know about?
_____

(Never leave this blank! Briefly include any volunteer work you've done with animals, any customer service experience, additional education, skills, or attributes you may have.)

Employment:

(If you have no paid employment but have volunteer work experience, fill this part out, stating your job title as volunteer and leave hourly pay rate blank. If you have more than three jobs, state the three most recent. If you have some paid and some volunteer work, list them in order of the dates, with the most recent first.)

(If you are an older student with years of work experience, the past ten years is all that is required. If you've been at the same job for the past ten years, you need only to put that one job, unless your other jobs were related to your current career or that you performed skills that would be beneficial in your current career.)

Always start with your most recent job and work back in reverse chronological order.

#1

Current or Most Recent Employer:_____

Address and Phone:_____

Job Title: _____ **Main Duties:**_____

Hourly Pay Rate:_____ **Dates of Employment:**_____

Reason for leaving:_____

(If your reason for leaving was less than favorable, you may or may not want to list it. It is not required to list a place of employment if you worked there less than six months to a year. Or you can state that it was simply "not a good fit." If you had to quit your job to concentrate on school, simple write, "School schedule." Never state anything negative on an application, no matter what! Do not say personal reasons!)

#2

Previous Employer:_____

Address and Phone:_____

Job Title: _____ **Main Duties:**_____

Hourly Pay Rate:_____ **Dates of Employment:**_____

Reason for leaving: _____

#3

Previous Employer_____

Address and Phone:_____

Job Title: _____ **Main Duties:**_____

Hourly Pay Rate:_____ **Dates of Employment:**_____

Reason for leaving:_____

Reference #1

Name:_____Relationship:_____

Phone: _____email: _____ How long have they know you?_____

Reference #2

Name:_____Relationship:_____

Phone: _____email: _____ How long have they know you?_____

Reference #3

Name:_____Relationship:_____

Phone: _____email: _____ How long have they know you?_____

Have you been convicted of a felony or misdemeanor or are presently/formally charged with committing any criminal offense? (Do not include any traffic violations, juvenile offenses, military convictions, except by general court martial.) If the answer is yes, furnish details of conviction, offense, location, date, and sentence. _____Yes _____No

I understand that any verbal or written statement that is false, fraudulent, or misleading that is contained in this application or attached materials, or made in the course of any related employment process, whether made by me or by others at my request, will result in rejection of my application, denial of employment, or dismissal from service if discovered after employment, and under some circumstances, may result in prosecution for a crime.

- I certify that all statements contained herein are true and complete.
- I understand that if hired, I must prove that I am legally authorized to work in the United States.
- I authorize the animal clinic to check employment references and verify education information provided on this employment application and as disclosed in the interview process.
- I authorize the animal clinic to run a credit history check and criminal history background check as a condition of employment.
- I release the animal clinic and all providers of information from any liability as a result of furnishing and receiving any information related to the hiring process.

Applicant Signature:_____

Constructing a Straightforward Winning Resume

Resume formats change every so often. Certain formats go in and out of style. But the order in which information is presented does not change. Be careful who you ask to review your resume. The person you ask might not be in the veterinary field, or even if they are, they may not have constructed a resume in many years and may not be familiar with the changes. Remember, you are not being hired on how creative and unique your resume looks in the veterinary field. Adding graphics or colored lines and a fancy font is not going to help you land the interview; it most likely will hurt your chances. Bullets are in and paragraphs are out when describing your work duties. Review the following before you begin writing your resume!

- *Do not* use an objective—just the title of the job you are applying for where the objective used to go—at the top of the page. After your name, email, address, and phone number, skip two lines.

- Education and employment are listed in reverse chronological order, with the *most recent first*, then the one right before that, the one before that, etc.

- Margins can go from .06 to one inch on all four sides. The top and bottom margins can be smaller than side margins.

- Use an easy-to-read font and size; font can go from eleven to twelve for the content, twelve to fourteen for headings.

- The best fonts for resumes are Cambria, Arial, Calibri, Verdana, Tacoma, Palatino, New Roman Times, Garamond, and Georgia.

- If you attended another school after high school and did not complete a degree, before attending your present school, type the name of the school, city, and state, and below that, approximately how many credits you completed and the dates that you attended—month/year only.

- *Do not* include your GPA (unless it is 3.5 or over)

- Never use all capital letters.

- Never use italics or underline or colons after headings.

- Spell out Street, Avenue, Lane, Road, and Court (in most cases)

- Abbreviate Twp., Blvd., Hwy., and Apt.

- Never use etc. on your resume.

- Use numbers for dates of employment: 05/15– 01/18 (in most cases)

- For states use postal codes (PA, OH, etc.)

- Bulleted duties or responsibilities need to be in the *past tense,* except for your current position (e.g., 02/17 – Present)

- Be consistent throughout your resume in spacing, indentations, bullets, and font.

- Bold headings. For example (only select the ones that pertain to you)

Your Name (only)	**Military Experience**	**Certifications**
Education	**Animal-Related Experience**	**Organizations**
Veterinary Technician	**Volunteer Work**	**Summary of Qualifications**
Veterinary Assistant	**Honors/Awards**	**Extracurricular Activities**
Work Experience	**Memberships**	**Computer Skills**

Be sure to have a professional-sounding email. If your current email is not a professional one, it is recommended that you open up a new account and use it just for your job search.

Jordan C. Brown

(Example 1—for those who have no paid work experience. Be sure to add spaces to spread out what you have on the page. If you were a member of any sports or clubs in high school, add those.)

jcb1001@gmail.com
602 Four Corners Road
Pittsburgh, PA 15777
724-676-8888

Veterinary Technician (or specific job title, if different than veterinary technician)

Education

Vet Tech Institute
Pittsburgh, PA
Associate Degree
Veterinary Technology
Graduating: 00/00

Pittsburgh Area High School
Pittsburgh, PA
High School Diploma
Track Team Member
Yearbook Committee
00/00

Volunteer Work

Animal Friends
Pittsburgh, PA
Dog Walker
00/00–00/00

Dianna M. Reid   (Example 2 for those who have had one paid work experience.)

diannamreid233@gmail.com
525 Penn Avenue
Pittsburgh, PA 15222
816-999-8989

Veterinary Technician (or specific job title, if different than veterinary technician)

Education

Vet Tech Institute, Pittsburgh, PA
Associate Degree in Veterinary Technology
Graduating: 00/00

South Side High School, Albany, NY
High School Diploma (or) GED Certificate
00/00

- Track and Field
- Field Hockey
- Key Club
- Marching Band, Choir, Band

Work Experience

Jake's Cafe, Albany, NY
00/00 -00/00
Customer Service

- Drive-through cashier
- Food prep
- Stock

(Example 3 for those who have attended another school prior to their present school, but did not complete a degree or certificate.)

Sara A. Beals

Saraabeals772@gmail.com

25 Hill Road
Toledo, OH 44700
330-233-2222

Veterinary Technician

(Or specific job title, if different than veterinary technician)

Education

Vet Tech Institute, Pittsburgh, PA	Graduating: 00/00
Associate Degree in Veterinary Technology	

Kent State University, Kent, OH	00/00–00/00
General Studies/Biology	
Completed 24 credits	

Hamburg High School, Toledo, OH	00/00
High School Diploma	
Marching Band	

Work Experience

First for Beauty, Pittsburgh, PA   00/00–Present
Sales Associate
- Educate customers on various beauty products
- Cashier duties

South Street Barbecue Company, Toledo, OH   00/00–00/00
Waitress/Hostess
- Waited tables
- Greeted customers
- Food preparation
- Cashier duties

Volunteer Work

Goodwill Industries Store, Toledo, OH   00/00–00/00
- Stocked shelves
- Unloaded shipments
- Cashier duties

(Example 4 for those who have completed another degree prior to attending their present school.)

Amanda L. Street

Alstreet121@yahoo.com

115 McKinney Street
Monroeville, PA 15002
724-999-7777

Veterinary Technician
(Or specific job title, if different than veterinary technician)

Education

Vet Tech Institute, Pittsburgh, PA
Associate Degree in Veterinary Technology
Graduating: 00/00

Waynesburg University, Waynesburg, PA
Bachelor of Science Degree, Biology
Graduated: 00/00

Bear Lake High School, Monroeville, PA
High School Diploma
Graduated: 00/00
National Honors Society, Volleyball, Softball

Work Experience

Olive Garden, Monroeville, PA
Server
- Serve food and sides
- Take food orders
- Interacting with the customers
- Cash out customers

00/00–Present

Five Guys Burgers and Fries, Monroeville, PA
Hostess and Cashier
- Cash out customers
- Take food orders

00/00–00/00

Volunteer Work

UPMC, Monroeville, PA
- Took test results and patient diagnostic request orders to the correct floors
- Escorting patients to their cars

00/00–00/00

Ashley A. Tremont

ashleyatreemont@yahoo.com

1234 High Point Drive
Pittsburgh, PA 15221
412-748-7777

Veterinary Technician

(Or specific job title, if different than veterinary technician)

Summary of Qualifications

Highly organized career changer with excellent communication and follow-through skills
Six years of volunteer work with the Humane Society of Western Pennsylvania
Lifelong animal lover

Education

Vet Tech Institute, Pittsburgh, PA	Graduating: 00/00
Associates Degree in Veterinary Technology	

University of North Carolina at Charlotte, Charlotte, NC	00/00
Bachelor of Arts, English Literature	

Employment

Trinity School for Ministry, Pittsburgh, PA	00/00–00/00

- Assistant Librarian

Sewickley Public Library, Pittsburgh, PA	00/00–00/00

- Clerk and Reference Assistant

Laughlin Memorial Public Library, Ambridge, PA	00/00–00/00

- Library Assistant

Dick Thornburgh Papers, University of Pittsburgh, Pittsburgh, PA	00/00–00/00

- Archival Assistant in the Service Center

Volunteer Work

Western Pennsylvania Humane Society, Pittsburgh, PA	00/00–Present

- Participate in various fundraising events
- Act as a "cat cuddler" on a biweekly basis
- Walk kennel dogs on a monthly basis

(Example 6 for those who have military experience)

Taylor Jameson

tjameson#33@gmail.com

234 Sidman Street
Pittsburgh, PA 15222
412-333-4456

Veterinary Technician

(Or specific job title, if different than veterinary technician)

Education

Vet Tech Institute, Pittsburgh, PA   Graduating: 00/00
Associate Degree in Veterinary Technology
Pennwood High School, Pennwood, PA   00/00
High School Diploma

- Swim team member
- National Honor Society

Work Experience

Camp Bow Wow, Pittsburgh, PA   00/00–Present
Doggie Day Care Attendant

- Feed and water dogs
- Supervise dogs in play yard
- Clean kennels

Military Experience

United States Navy, USS Gravely DDG 100, Norfolk, VA   00/00–00/00
Interior Communications Electrician

Fireman Recruit, Fireman, Great Lakes, IL and Norfolk, VA   00/00–00/00
Pre-commissioning Destroyer Unit

Volunteer Work

Humane Society of Norfolk, Norfolk, VA   00/00–00/00

- Fed animals
- Medicated animals
- Cleaned dog and cat kennels

Reference Page—Sample

Name
Email
Street Address
City, State Zip Code
Phone

References

Howard Isenberg, D.V.M.
Robert L. Lash Veterinary Associates
170 East Brady Road
Kittanning, PA 16201
724-543-2814
Email

Jessica Todd
Head Vet Tech
East McKeesport Pet Hospital
11 Lincoln Highway
North Versailles, PA 15111
412-901-4333
Email

Renae Smith
Head Cashier
Save Mart
226 Tenth Street
Erie, PA 16506
814-570-0693
Email

Very important—you need to ask permission to use someone as a reference. Explain to them what type of position you are applying for and that they may be getting a phone call in the future.

People who could be references: Current or former employers, teachers, volunteer supervisors, and organization, club, or church group leaders.

*Do **not** use as a reference:* Family members, friends, boyfriends, girlfriends, boyfriends' or girlfriends' parents, classmates, or employers who were less than satisfied with your work or where you left on questionable terms.

- The heading on your reference page should match the heading on your resume, with the same font and font size. *Single space* reference information, and *double space* between references.

- There should be a one-inch margin on the top and sides.

- Bold only your *name* and the title *"References."*

Letters of Recommendation and Reference Letters

The person who writes a letter of recommendation knows the candidate well enough to evaluate his or her abilities.

A letter of recommendation is generally requested by the candidate for a particular career goal, academic application, or job opportunity. The letter details the candidate's accomplishments and skills that make him or her a strong contender and is based on the writer's personal experience with this candidate. Also, a letter of recommendation, which is addressed to a specific recipient, is stronger than a reference letter because the writer is actually recommending you for a job.

A letter of recommendation is preferred for professional jobs. This letter is most often written by one of the people listed on your reference page. This person knows you well, but when you ask someone to write a letter of recommendation, it's best to give the writer details about what type of job you are looking for and what skills are needed in that job. When you accept a position, be sure to inform the person who took the time and made an effort to construct a letter for you. If you do not have a person in your life who can write about you in some detail for an employer, a reference letter is your next best tool.

A reference letter is more general in nature. Typically, it is not addressed to an individual.

A letter of reference is an overall assessment of the candidate's characteristics, knowledge, and skills. Context of how the writer knows the individual is included, such as, "I was Clara's supervisor at Don's Pet Supplies." In some cases, a company representative will issue a letter of reference that simply states the former employee's dates of employment and job title. This letter merely references that the writer knows you and confirms basic facts about you. A reference letter is a valuable tool when it comes to your job search. Do not minimize the positive impact it will have on future employers.

Why Letters Written about You are Important to Employers

When a person in your life (a former employer, teacher, scout leader, pastor, or coach) thinks enough of you to spend the time writing a letter on your behalf, it means a great deal to a potential employer. A thoughtful letter means much more that a verbal recommendation or reference. Responding to a phone call does not require the effort that a letter requires.

Many employers request recommendation letters to help them make hiring decisions. Throughout the hiring process, applicants strive to present themselves in the best light. Beyond the interview and resume, hiring managers look to recommendation letters to *confirm the candidate's qualifications and to gain insight from an outside party.*

The hiring manager wants to know what experiences the candidate will bring to the new role, how he or she will contribute to the company, and how the applicant will behave day to day. Recommendation letters can *point to a candidate's future performance by talking about past achievements.*

Reference letters can also shed light on the duties or work performance of an individual and confirm that the person worked for the employer at a particular time. Reference letters are more general but are also worthwhile to provide to a future employer.

The ideal letter should be written to "Dear Future Employer." It should be typed on the letterhead of the company, school, or organization of the person writing the letter and should explain how the person knows you. It should be signed in ink by the person writing the letter.

The following are acceptable:

- The letter is emailed to you with a typed signature.

- The letter is not on letterhead.

- A letter that was written as a requirement for admission to a veterinary nurse/technician program.

  If the interviewer asks, "What would your references say about you?" you can answer with information that was in your letter of reference/recommendation.

Creating a Career Portfolio

IT'S A PROCESS

The most important benefit to creating a career portfolio is that it develops an orderly mind-set of what you will need to present about yourself to an employer. The time and effort you put into portfolio development is a true investment in your career. The process of examining your skills, abilities, achievements, and weaknesses can build confidence, so there is little or nothing an interviewer can ask that you haven't already thought about.

IT'S PROOF

Instead of just talking about what you can do during an interview or job review, you can show the interviewer your portfolio, filled with achievements, awards, letters of recommendation, and pictures of your successful interactions with clients, staff, classmates, and animals.

STAND OUT AND INTERVIEW WITH CONFIDENCE

A career portfolio is a record of your education, work, and volunteer experiences that you can take with you on a job interview. Your portfolio will be *customized* to show pictures of you working with animals, working as part of a team, or participating in something that is unique or noteworthy. It should include certificates you have earned or honors you have achieved.

Developing a portfolio will help you get organized and prepared for the job market. It also serves as a great tool in an interview (especially if you have difficultly talking about yourself). Having a neat, well-organized portfolio also projects a professional image.

RESEARCH, RESEARCH, RESEARCH

It is essential to know something about the clinic, hospital, or research facility before you go on an externship/internship or job interview.

There are several ways to select where you want to complete an externship or secure a job in the veterinary industry. You can talk to former students who now work at a particular site, ask your teachers, or contact people you know who are clients at the hospital or clinic near where you live.

What if you are not familiar with the area where you are planning to live after you complete your schooling? If you have no idea what is in your area, or even if you do, the first step is to visit the websites of potential employers.

Many interviewers will ask you what you know about their facility. If you cannot respond to this question, you most likely will not be considered for a job or an externship there.

Gather the following information, put it in your portfolio, and bring it to the interview so you can review important information about the site.

Use your favorite search engine on your computer:

- Type in **Veterinary Hospitals** and the **City** and **State** of where you are considering doing an externship.
- Scroll down. A list will come up.
- Review the websites of the various hospitals or clinics and determine if they offer the services and environment that interests you.
- Select one that most interests you, and another as a back- up.
- Gather the following information for your portfolio.

1. Full name of clinic or hospital
2. Full address
3. Telephone number
4. Fax number (you may need to call the facility for this)
5. Email address (you may need to call the facility for this)
6. Website address (you may need to call the clinic)
7. Name of the practice manager, office manager, head technician, or veterinarian
8. What kind of practice it is: emergency, mixed, large animal, etc.
9. The *main* services that they provide
10. Something *unique* about the clinic

Type the above information on a separate sheet of paper and place it in your portfolio. You may want to include more information from the clinic's website. Review this sheet before your interview.

Contents of Your Career Portfolio

You do not need to purchase an expensive leather portfolio to take on an interview. A three-ring, one-inch black, dark blue, or maroon binder with a front sleeve is sufficient. Non-glare plastic sheet protectors for the contents are recommended.

Professional and tasteful portfolio cover (with your name)

Suggestions for the cover are picture(s) of your animals, you working with animals, the vet tech oath, or a saying about animals. It's a great icebreaker in an interview.

1. **Your resume (two copies)**

   Put one in plastic and one in the *front* portfolio pocket, to be given to the interviewer if he or she does not have your current resume.

2. **Your references (two copies)**

   Put one in plastic and one in the *back* pocket of the portfolio.

3. **At least one letter of recommendation**

   This should be from your present or former employer, volunteer coordinator, or former instructor/professor.

4. **Awards/certificates**

   Include achievements at your place of employment or where you have done volunteer work or an honor roll or attendance award from your educational institution. If you do not have an actual certificate, but you do have volunteer activities, list those activities.

5. **Pictures**

   Arrange the photos on paper: you working or participating as part of a team—with or without animals—your animals, you with your animals, you interacting with your animals or other animals (showing or performing, for example). Color photos are preferred, but black and white is acceptable.

The following items need to be in your portfolio to keep you organized for the interview. They are NOT to be shown to the interviewer. Add a divider sheet of paper, (other than white) to keep these items separate, from the items to be shown to the interviewer!

- Include your sample job application, so you can copy it onto their application if asked.

- Have the research on where you are interviewing, including the name of the interviewer, available for your reference.

- Write a list of questions to ask the interviewer.

- Include sample interview questions with your answers to review.

- Write a thank-you card or letter with an envelope addressed to where you are interviewing and a stamp, so you can send your thank-you letter as soon as you complete it following the interview.

The number of pages in your portfolio depends on your opportunities, level of achievement, and—in many cases—your age. Remember, your portfolio is a process and a way to organize yourself for the interview. A number of candidates do not have awards or volunteer experiences to put in their portfolios. After putting your portfolio together, you may want to consider volunteering with animals or seeking out additional letters of recommendation prior to your actual job search.

If your school requires an internship or externship, you can use that setting to add achievements to your portfolio. Ask for a letter of recommendation from the supervisor at your internship or externship, just prior to completing all your requirements. Students often find it much more difficult to secure letters of recommendation once they leave the work site after completing their internship or externship.

Externships vs. Internships! What Is the Difference?

EXTERNSHIPS

An externship in the field of veterinary care support usually takes place the final term of the program, prior to graduation. All course work has been completed. Externships are typically not paid, but on occasion they can be, depending on the facility. The actual number of hours that the student works is determined by the school. There is an exchange of services for experience between the extern and the facility. In many instances a contract is signed by the school and the facility with specific skills outlined and signed off by the veterinarian, or the designated supervisor of the externs. School credit is given for this experience, and an evaluation of the student's performance on the externship is provided by a designated person at the externship site.

Providing a hands-on experience for students benefits the employer due to the fact that the extern is familiar with the staff and the routine of the facility and cuts down on the time it takes to train a new employee. It is also beneficial to the student due to the fact that they have the opportunity to adjust to the facility's routine and staff and become comfortable with the environment. Their period of being "new" is already completed.

An externship is a win-win for employers who are looking to hire and students who are seeking a job! However, there is no guarantee of a job following an externship, and there is no obligation to hire an extern following completion of the externship hours.

A less-than-positive experience at a particular externship site can actually benefit the student as well as the employer. The student learns that their personality does not mesh with the other staff members, or that they are not in agreement with certain practices and policies or that the duties that they are asked to perform are not the ones that the student is most interested in doing as a full-time job. *Finding out what you don't want do is a valuable lesson, and it prevents you pursuing a path that you may have thought you wanted but have now found out that you need to look in another direction.*

The employer benefits because they find out that the extern is not a good fit, and they can then pursue someone who will be more successful working in their facility.

INTERNSHIPS

Internships and externships often have the same requirements in the field of veterinary care support. It is just a matter of what word a particular school uses. In some schools students work at their internship two to three days a week and attend classes the other days. At times internships are paid and conducted during a school break, not at the end of the degree program. Internships may or may not be paid. Internships may or may not be required. Career schools that teach skills for specific employment opportunities require internships or externships. It is wise to clarify what your specific school requires prior to beginning your program of study.

Both externships and internships provide students the ability to receive hands-on learning about a particular future career, preparing them for full-time work following graduation.

Cover Letter Example for a Student Seeking an Externship/Internship in the Veterinary Care Industry

(*If you are emailing* your resume, type in the subject line, "Externship Possibility." Then attach your cover letter and resume in two separate documents. Name your documents, "Last name, First Name, Cover Letter," and "Last Name, First Name Resume.")

Date

Dr. Brian Pettigrew
City Veterinary Hospital
12 S. Main Street
Canton, OH 43506

Dear Dr. Pettigrew:

I am presently a student at _____(name of school, city, and state) and am very interested in securing an externship at _____ (name facility).

While researching (or touring) your facility, I very much liked the fact that_____ (for example: you also treat exotics, which are a particular interest of mine).

The externship is a requirement for _____. This degree program is accredited by the AVMA, which allows all graduates to sit for the licensing exam.

The externship consists of working in an animal hospital for a total of _____ hours throughout a(an) _____ week term beginning _____ and ending _____.

Although the externship does not begin until _____, (date) _____ (name of school) requires that we secure our externship site and have all required paperwork completed and filed approximately six weeks prior to the start of the externships, which is _____ (date).

An externship packet detailing the requirement will be sent to you by _____ once you indicated your interest in participating in our externship program. (Include the procedure that your particular school requires.)

I will make the necessary arrangements to speak with you in person or on the telephone about my qualifications for the externship. I have attached my resume for your review.

Sincerely,

Sign your name

Type your first and last name
Phone number
Email

Cover Letter Example for a Graduate Seeking a Job in the Veterinary Care Industry

(If you are emailing your resume, type in the subject line the name of the job that you are apply for "Veterinary Technician Position." Then attach your cover letter and resume in two separate documents. Name your documents, "Last name, First Name, Cover Letter," and "Last Name, First Name Resume.")*

Date

John Smith, DVM
Scottsdale Animal Clinic
222 Amber Way
Scottsdale, AZ 34345

Dear Dr. Smith,

I am very interested in the _____ position at the Humane Society, which I saw advertised on your website.

I am a recent graduate of _____ and have always been interested in working in a shelter setting. I feel that my heart and my skills are best suited for working within this type of environment. I completed a (an) _____ week externship/internship with _____ and was given the opportunity to practice a number of the skills I learned in school, _____.

As you can see by my enclosed (or attached) resume, I also have customer service experience while working in the retail industry while in high school and during weekends while completing my associate's degree.

I look forward to the opportunity to speak with you about my experience and qualifications for the job.

Sincerely,

Sign your name

Type your name
Type your phone number
Email

Adding Your Externship or Internship to Your Resume

There are a few different ways you can add your externship or internship to your resume. The most logical place, in my professional opinion, is under the heading "Education" and under the school in which you graduated and earned credits for completing your externship or internship. Add a few of the main skills that you practiced on your externship or internship. Be sure to put the most notable veterinary care skills that you did first and incidental tasks that you were required to do, such as cleaning kennels or answering phones. Do not list everything you did. It takes up too much room on your one-page resume as well as leaving little to talk about on an interview concerning your externship or internship.

For example:

Education

Vet Tech Institute, Pittsburgh, PA   00/00

Associate Degree in Veterinary Technology

    Externship: _____*(required hours completed)*   00/00–00/00

    Northside Veterinary Clinic, Pittsburgh, PA

    Main skills practiced:

- Placed catheters; took x-rays
- Administered vaccines; restrained animals; pre- and post-surgery duties
- Greeted clients; took patient histories; front desk duties

In some cases students were already employed, in some capacity, at their externship/internship site prior to starting to work the hours that were evaluated for credit at their school. In this case the externship can go under "Work Experience" and your job title would be Extern or Intern.

For example:

Education

Vet Tech Institute, Pittsburgh, PA   00/00
Associate Degree in Veterinary Technology

Southside High School, Pittsburgh, PA   00/00
High School Diploma

Work Experience

Northside Veterinary Clinic, Pittsburgh, PA
Extern   00/00–00/00
Main skills practiced:
  • Placed catheters; took x-rays
  • Administered vaccines; restrained animals; pre- and post-surgery duties
  • Greeted clients; took patient histories; front desk duties
Kennel Assistant   00/00–00/00
  • Walked kennel dogs
  • Fed dogs and cats
  • Cleaned kennels

If you have other animal-related experience at a different facility than your externship site, you can also put your externship under "Work Experience." Your title will be "Extern."

For Example:

Education

Vet Tech Institute, Pittsburgh, PA   00/00

Associate Degree in Veterinary Technology

Southside High School, Pittsburgh, PA   00/00
High School Diploma

Work Experience

Northside Veterinary Clinic, Pittsburgh, PA

Extern: 270 Hours   00/00–00/00

- Placed catheters; took x-rays
- Administered vaccines; restrained animals; pre- and post-surgery duties
- Greeted clients; took patient histories; front desk duties

West End Animal Hospital, Westfield, NY   00/00–00/00

Kennel Assistant

- Walked kennel dogs
- Fed dogs and cats
- Cleaned kennels

Dog Stop Doggie Day Care, West Field, NY   00/00–00/00

Attendant

- Interacted with dogs at play time at the day care
- Fed dogs according owners' instructions

Updating Your Resume after Working at a Job in Your Field of Choice!

You are probably excited and a bit overwhelmed by your new responsibilities and the new people, and you will be working and relieved that you no longer need to job search. But within a month or following your probation period in your new position, it is best to update your resume with your new job! Once you are working in the field that you prepared for in school, the format of your resume changes. The heading "Work Experience" replaces the "Education" heading at the top of your resume. You will now want to emphasize *your work experience* rather than *your education* once you are employed in the field.

The heading "Education" goes at the *bottom* of your resume after you start to working in the field of your choice. It is also important to add certified, registered, or licensed (depending on where you live) to veterinary technician if you have graduated from a school that allows you to sit for the Veterinary Technician National Exam (VTNE). You no longer need to include bulleted items for your current position unless you perform a unique service that other veterinary technicians do not normally do in the course of their work day. If your former jobs are not self-explanatory, then you do not need to elaborate on your duties. If you earn continuing education credits, you may want to take your high school off of your resume, if you need more space, or if it's been over ten years since you graduated.

Amanda L. Street

Alstreet121@yahoo.com

115 McKinney Street

Monroeville, PA 15002

724-999-7777

Certified Veterinary Technician

Work Experience

County Veterinary Hospital, Pittsburgh, PA	00/00–00/00
Certified Veterinary Technician	

Steel City Veterinary Clinic, Pittsburgh, PA	00/00–00/00
Kennel Assistant	

Olive Garden, Monroeville, PA	00/00–00/00
Server	

Five Guys Burgers and Fries, Monroeville, PA	00/00–00/00
Hostess and Cashier	

Volunteer Work

UPMC, Monroeville, PA   00/00–00/00
- Took test results and patient diagnostic request orders to the correct floors
- Escorted patients to their cars

Education

Vet Tech Institute, Pittsburgh, PA	00/00
Associate Degree in Veterinary Technology	
Northside Veterinary Clinic, Pittsburgh, PA	00/00–00/00
Extern: 270 Hours	

Bear Lake High School, Monroeville, PA	00/00–00/00
High School Diploma	

National Honors Society, Volleyball, Softball

Thank-You Notes or Letters after the Interview

The thank-you note or letter is still an essential part of the interview process.

A thank-you note does the following.

1. **It expresses your interest in the position.**

   During the interview process, everything from your tone to word choice should express a sincere interest in working at that organization. However, some of those signals may have been missed by the interviewer or you may have been exhausted by the time you reached the final interview segment. A thank-you note is your opportunity to reaffirm your interest in the position.

2. **It shows you have manners.**

   Yes, your grandmother was right about manners. They do matter. In the working world after meeting with a customer or partner, it is essential to follow up with him or her. Sending a thank-you note after your interview is an indicator that you already have the skills to properly represent an organization.

3. **It can tip the scale in your favor.**

   A few hours in an interview does not provide the insight that working with someone for a few months can provide. For that reason, most interviewers are not 100 percent certain of which candidate to hire. Often at the end of the process, it is a toss-up between the top two candidates. A thank-you note can be the tiebreaker.

When writing a thank you note, keep these things in mind.

- **Keep it brief.**

  It essential to express your interest in the position. However, that does not mean you need to write an essay on the topic. Limit your note to a few paragraphs. Keep in mind that interviewing candidates is typically done in addition to an interviewer's normal work. Be considerate of his or her time.

- **Write a note for each interviewer.**

  It takes more time to write a note for each interviewer. However, it is worth the extra time. Keep in mind that they are likely to see each other's notes, so make each note a bit different. To prepare for the note writing, at the end of each interview segment, ask the interviewers for their business cards (if you do not already have their contact information).

- **Clarify your answers.**

  Did you stumble on a question during the interview? A thank-you note can be your opportunity to fix that blunder. Use a couple of sentences to give some additional insight into your answer.

Thank-You Letter Example

(A *plain* white or cream-colored thank-you card that is handwritten is a nice touch, but be sure your handwriting is neat and legible. If it is not, type a letter and put it into a thank-you card. A typed letter that is mailed or emailed is acceptable. The *timing* of sending a thank-you letter after an interview is important. Send your thank you the *same day* as your interview to make the most impact, especially if the interviewer had several candidates to interview.)

Date

Name
Title of Interviewer
Name of Veterinary Hospital or Clinic, etc.
Street address
City, State zip code

Dear Mr. Archer:

Thank you for taking the time to interview me on _____. It was a pleasure meeting you and discussing my qualifications for the _____ (specific job title) opening at your _____ Veterinary Hospital.

After _____ (point out something about the facility that impressed you, for example, the type of equipment, the staff, etc.), I am even more excited about the possibility of working for _____ (add name of the hospital). I wanted to add that I am also interested in _____ (add something you may have forgotten to say on the interview—for example, you like exotics and have owned tree frogs and a boa constrictor for the past several years).

I look forward to hearing from you.

Sincerely,

Sign your name
Phone number
Email

ALL ABOUT
THE INTERVIEW

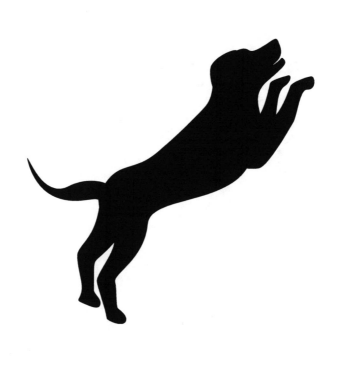

The Real Point of an Interview

Interviews aren't as concerned with each individual answer as much as how you present them and *the total picture* they help paint of you. While of course each answer goes into creating the picture, there's so much more to doing well in an interview.

Interviewers want to see the whole package. Although not every interviewer looks for the same thing, in general they are looking for things like, but not limited to, the following:

- An ability to tell your story in a way that presents you in a positive light
- What would you be like to work with on a daily basis
- Your attitude during the entire interview process
- Whether you see things as problems or challenges
- Skills that you know how to apply in the real-world workplace
- Willingness to learn new things
- Willingness to take on problems and solve them
- Knowing how and when to involve others in those solutions
- Ability to communicate with clients as well as coworkers and supervisors
- Ability to work with people—especially with different points of view and ages
- Evidence that you understand work is mainly about the employer's needs and not just about your individual needs and preferences
- Lack of potential problems (are you low maintenance?) and *no drama*
- Reliability in terms of transportation and weather issues

While your individual answers go into the impression you make, it's not just the words that matter. It's also about how you present the words and how you present yourself, as well as whether the interviewer got to see the real person or canned answers you thought he or she wanted to hear.

Spend time preparing stories about your work history that show why you are great for *this* particular job! Practice talking about yourself and your previous jobs in a natural manner so the interviewer can see the very best of who you really are.

The bottom line is that *every* question interviewers ask you is to find out the following:

- Will you do what they want you to do the way they want you to do it?

- Will you get along with others at work, including employees and clients?

- Will you show up on time, do your work, leave any problems at home, and cause no drama at work?

- Will you represent them well through your actions, communication, and appearance?

Write Your Own Want Ad!

You will be interviewing a person to care for your beloved ten-year-old dog, who suffers from diabetes and arthritis. You need someone you trust and who will be able to give your dog medications (injections and pills) and also take your dog on two slow twenty-minute walks a day. State the days, dates, and time they will be needed throughout this five-day job. Include what you will need from them in terms of references, and/or a resume or if you just want to meet with them. Also include how they are to contact you. You can include the rate of payment per day in your ad if you want.

What skills and characteristics will you want this person to have, and who will respond to your ad? Will you require experience and/or a certain educational level for this candidate? Be complete. Write this ad as if you were going to post it on the internet or on a local bulletin board.

_____

_____

_____

_____

_____

_____

_____

_____

_____

_____

_____

_____

_____

_____

_____

_____

_____

_____

_____

_____

_____

_____

WHAT EMPLOYERS ARE LOOKING FOR WHEN HIRING IN THE VETERINARY CARE FIELD

Employers are looking for individuals with a *will-do* attitude. They are looking for a person who is willing to learn the procedures of the particular facility, even if they have learned a different way, while attending school or working in another facility. A positive attitude and a willingness to learn is what employers want in an employee, but they also want someone who has the capability, education, and experiences that prove that he or she *can do* the job.

Use the following lists as a guide when preparing to answer interview questions. Give examples of how you possess as many of these characteristics as you can when completing the worksheets in this book.

ATTITUDES (WILL DO)

- **Initiative**: A person with initiative shows willingness and aptitude to take appropriate steps in finding solutions to problems and presents options and ideas to enhance current processes or procedures. He or she takes an additional responsibility when both big and small tasks need to be done.

- **Integrity:** A person with integrity firmly adheres to the values and ethics of the facility. He or she exhibits honesty, discretion, and sound judgment.

- **Cooperativeness**: A person who is cooperative is willing to work with others, collaborating and compromising where necessary, and promptly shares relevant information with others.

- **Flexibility:** Someone with flexibility is open to changing situations and opportunities and is willing to perform all tasks assigned.

- **Independence:** A person who is independent is able and willing to perform tasks and duties without supervision as appropriate.

- **Tolerance for Stress/Resiliency:** A person with this characteristic maintains a positive can-do outlook, rebounds quickly from frustrations and unpleasantness, and maintains composure and a friendly demeanor while dealing with stressful situations.

CAPABILITIES, EDUCATION AND EXPERIENCE (CAN DO)

- **Communication Skills:** Someone with communication skills reads, writes, and speaks fluent English, using appropriate grammar, style, and vocabulary. He or she correctly spells commonly used English words and job-specific terms. He or she demonstrates exceptionally strong written and verbal communication skills.

- **Organizational Ability:** One with organizational ability demonstrates a systematic approach in carrying out assignments. He or she is very orderly and excels at cutting through confusion and turning chaos into order.

- **Problem-Solving Skills:** Someone with problem-solving skills demonstrates a strong ability to identify, analyze, and solve problems and translates problems into practical solutions.

- **Client Service Skills:** People with client service skills consistently make sure that the team provides clients with attentive, courteous, and informative service. They show personal satisfaction after delivering great service.

- **Intellectual Ability:** People with intellectual ability accurately and consistently follow instructions delivered in an oral, written, or diagram format. They can provide directions.

- **Ability to Multitask:** These people can manage multiple tasks at one time. They quickly and accurately shift their attention among multiple tasks under distracting conditions without loss of accuracy or the appearance of frustration.

- **Mathematical Ability:** These people have the ability to add, subtract, multiply, and divide, and to compute rate, ratio, and percent. They also have the ability to convert units of measurement.

- **Computer Skills:** Those with computer skills can comfortably and confidently use a computer and specialized software.

Behavioral Interviewing

S.T.A.R

Situation

Task

Action

Result

- With the *S* portion of STAR, you are focusing first on a *situation*. When interviewers pose a question to you, they generally want the most crucial information that you have, not the fluffy stuff. You are basically setting the stage to answering an often-boring question with a notable and unforgettable response.

- Following the stage-setting S portion of the STAR interviewing process comes the *T*. In this acronym, T stands for task. Once you've led with what the background situation was, you need to show what *task* was needed to handle that circumstance. Describing the task that needed to be completed shows the interviewer exact challenges that you faced to handle the situation you listed above.

- After laying down the task at hand, it's time to show the *action* that you took, or the *A* portion. This is where you explain exactly how you went about tackling that circumstance and what skills and talents of yours that it took to do so.

- Last but not least, you have the *R: result*. It is possibly the most informative portion of the STAR interviewing technique. Make sure you end with a bang by highlighting your result. *Be specific!*

Common Behavioral Interview Questions

Describe a time when you had to interact with a difficult customer or client or just another person in your life. What was the situation, and how did you handle it?

How will the interviewer remember you?

Write a paragraph about what is *unique* about you. What would make you stand out to an employer so that they would remember you after interviewing many candidates? Remember, *not too personal*. It should be something you could tell an employer.

What is a special skill you have (that would help in your vet tech career)?

Do you have a volunteer experience that will help you in your career?

What is an accomplishment that you are proud of?

Talk about a trip that you took—out of the country perhaps. What did you learn or discover about yourself?

What is an event in your life that changed you for the better in some way?

Talk about an animal you helped in some way, whether you adopted, rehabilitated, or saved it.

_____

_____

_____

_____

_____

_____

_____

_____

_____

_____

_____

_____

_____

_____

_____

What would you consider your greatest weakness (challenge)?

This is definitely a popular question that is asked by interviewers.

While *weakness* is a harsh word, remember that nobody is perfect, and we all have areas of development that we need to work on.

Employers understand this and ask the question for two reasons.

- First, they want to make sure your weakness isn't a skill they need someone to have mastery of immediately (basic vet tech skills, math ability, patience, or inability to control your emotions, for example).
- Second, they want to see how you handle yourself under pressure and when asked tough questions.

We advise our candidates to be honest and focus on a weakness that is not one of the top qualities or skills required for the job.

Also, be sure to describe how you've already taken steps and made strides in strengthening this skill, showing your ability and desire to constantly learn and grow.

THE BOTTOM LINE

Interviewers want to make certain that they don't have to worry about you as an employee. You need to assure them that you will be a good employee and there will be no reason to worry!

This question is reported to be one of the most difficult questions to answer on an interview.

Some suggestions on how to answer the question of a weakness or a challenge that you have faced follow.

1. I used to be a bit scattered and unorganized in my study habits in high school, although I got good grades. (Make sure this is true for you.) I didn't really need to be that organized to do well. Once I started at _____ (name of current school), I had to develop a system of note taking and set aside certain times of the evening to study certain subjects, which I did. (Describe how this has helped you.) This has helped me a great deal.

2. I tend to be a bit shy, so I when I started on the path to my new career, I made an extra effort to speak up in class, ask questions, and try to start conversations with my classmates. Although it's still a bit difficult, I've come a long way and know that I can handle speaking with new people in a clinic setting.

3. My weakness was dealing with reptiles, especially snakes. We had a guest speaker in class who brought in some of her pets, which included several different types of snakes and an iguana. I made myself hold each one and got a bit more used to them. The snakes were actually beautiful creatures, and although they are not my favorites, by far, I do not fear holding them any longer.

The key is to be honest and sincere without being negative and worrisome to an employer!

Questions Not to Ask
on an Interview

Most of these questions you can ask *after* you are offered the position. Do not ask these at all during an interview.

1. What is the pay for this position?
2. Do you offer health benefits? What does that include?
3. Is there vacation during the first year of employment?
4. Do your employees get along?
5. What is your policy on convenience euthanasia?
6. Do you *pay* for CE credits?
7. Do I *have* to work overtime often?
8. Will I be working *every* weekend?
9. Where did you go to school to become a tech? Are you certified?
10. Is this an AHHA certified hospital?
11. Is there room for advancement? (When you are first out of school and interviewing for your first vet tech job, the employer wants to hire a tech. They don't want to hire someone who will want to take over and who has a great deal of ambition to move on. If you ask this question, you probably won't be hired at anywhere other than a large emergency clinic that does have room for advancement. Although you won't need to ask that on an interview, you will already know that from your research.)

---

*Always remember that on the interview you are there to describe what **you**
can offer an employer, not what an employer can offer you!*

Once you are offered the position, you can ask any question on this list in a professional manner. Instead of asking if whoever interviewed you is a certified tech, you can ask how many certified techs they employ and how many are not certified.

After you are offered the position, this is *what you need to know* before you start your first shift!

- Your pay and benefits
- Date and time you are to start
- The dress code and what you should wear your first day
- What your schedule is for the week you begin

Some suggested questions that you should ask the interviewer on the interview!

- What qualities are you looking for in a new hire?

- Are you adding or replacing an employee?

- Can you describe a typical day in your clinic/hospital?

- What do you believe to be the main challenges of a new hire?

- Can you tell me about the team I'd be working with?

- Do you have a formal training program for new hires?

- How would my performance be evaluated? How often?

- Is there a probationary period for new hires? If so, how long is it?

- Who would I report to directly?

- How long have you worked here?

- What is your favorite part of working here?

- Is there anything you'd like me to do before you make a decision?

- Can I have a tour of the building?

- Do you need anything else from me (like my references or to job shadow)?

- What is the next step in the hiring process?

- Should I call or email you, or will you be notifying me either way?

- When do you expect to be making a hiring decision? When would you like the new hire to start to work?

Select three or four questions that have not already been answered in the interview. Never leave an interview without knowing when and if you will be notified about their decision!

Popular Interview Questions in the Veterinary Care Field

No negative answers!

To be most effective in preparing for the interview, it is suggested that you write or type out the answers to each of these questions, take them on the interview with you, and review them before going into the interview.

1. Tell me about yourself. (Do not share personal information, such as you age or your relationship status.)

    Hint: Tell the interviewer why you decided to become a vet tech and why you selected the school you went to, especially if you are not from this area. Name a couple of your favorite classes and why you liked them. Let the interviewer know some of the positive characteristics you have that will make you a great vet tech, as well as some of the skills that you have learned at school.

2. What is your greatest strength?

    Hint: Name only one and explain why that is your greatest strength. Give an example of how you can demonstrate that you have this strength.

3. What is a weakness or challenge that you have, and *what steps you have been taking to improve or overcome this?*

    Hint: *Do not* name a basic veterinary care skill or requirement (i.e., restraining or math). *Do not* say that you are a perfectionist. The interviewer may worry that you'll be too slow, double checking your work.

4. What would your references say about you?

    Hint: Answer with something that is written in your letter of recommendation. If you don't have a letter, then name one or two *specific* things that a reference has said or would tell an employer about you. (Just saying they would say all good things is not enough!)

5. Where do you see yourself in five years?

    Hint: Do not talk about your long-term plans. Just say that you will be a certified technician who is more skilled and confident in the profession. This answer should reflect long-term interest in staying at the place that you interview, so they will feel that you are worth putting the time and training into you as a tech.

6. Do you have any questions for me?

   Hint: Refer to "Question You Should Ask on an Interview" and "Questions *Not* to Ask on an Interview."

7. Why should I hire you over other candidates?

   Hint: The interviewer does not want you to actually try and compare yourself to anyone else. They want to hear what strengths and skills that *you* would bring to the job. Do not put down classmates or coworkers in your answer.

Be Prepared to Answer These Additional Interview Questions

Tell me about a time that you made a mistake and what you did about it.

Explain the reasons why all dogs should be on heartworm preventative and what the procedure is for this (as if you are speaking with a new client).

_____

_____

_____

_____

_____

_____

_____

_____

_____

_____

_____

_____

_____

_____

_____

_____

_____

_____

_____

_____

_____

_____

_____

_____

_____

_____

_____

_____

_____

_____

_____

_____

_____

_____

1. What job did you like best? What job did you like least? Why? If you haven't had many jobs, what *duties* did you like best? Least? Why?

_____

_____

_____

_____

2. Why do you want to work for this practice? Why do you think you would fit in here?

_____

_____

_____

_____

3. Tell me about a time that you had to resolve a conflict. What was the situation, and how did you handle it? What was the outcome?

_____

_____

_____

_____

4. Tell me about a time where you had to adapt quickly to an adverse event or situation.

_____

_____

_____

_____

5. Tell me about a time when you had to work with someone very challenging to work with and how you dealt with the situation.

_____

_____

_____

_____

Fifty Most Common Job Interview Mistakes

1. Arriving late

2. Arriving too early (Fifteen minutes early is sufficient. The interviewer may feel pressured if you are too early.)

3. Smelling like a cigarette or alcohol

4. Bad-mouthing your last boss or teacher, or classmate, or anyone

5. Lying about your skills, experiences, and knowledge

6. Wearing the wrong clothes

7. Forgetting the name of the person you are interviewing with

8. Wearing a ton of perfume or aftershave

9. Wearing sunglasses

10. Wearing a Bluetooth earpiece

11. Failing to research the employer in advance

12. Failing to demonstrate enthusiasm

13. Inquiring about benefits before being offered the job

14. Asking about salary before being offered the job

15. Being unable to explain how your strengths, experience, and abilities apply to this job

16. Failing to make a strong case for why you are the best person for this job

17. Forgetting to bring a copy of your resume and/or portfolio

18. Failing to remember what you wrote on your own resume

19. Asking too many questions

20. Asking no questions at all

21. Being unprepared to answer the standard questions

22. Failing to listen carefully to what the interviewer is saying

23. Talking more than half of the time

24. Interrupting your interviewer

25. Neglecting to match the communication style of your interviewer (voice volume)

26. Yawning

27. Slouching

28. Bringing along a friend, or your mother or dad

29. Chewing gum, tobacco, your pen, or your hair

30. Laughing, giggling, leg jiggling, pen clicking, swiveling in your chair

31. Saying "you know," "like," "I guess," and "um" or "so" and "well" (before answering each question)

32. Name-dropping or bragging or sounding like a know-it-all

33. Asking to use the bathroom (during the interview)

34. Being falsely or exaggeratedly modest (if you are complimented on *anything*, say thank you)

35. Shaking hands too weakly

36. Failing to make eye contact (or making continuous eye contact, staring)

37. Taking a seat before your interviewer does

38. Becoming angry or defensive

39. Complaining that you were kept waiting

40. Complaining about anything!

41. Speaking rudely to the receptionist (You are being evaluated as soon as you walk in the door.)

42. Letting your nervousness show

43. Overexplaining why you lost your last job

44. Being too familiar and jokey

45. Sounding desperate

46. Checking the time

47. Oversharing

48. Sounding rehearsed

49. Leaving your cell phone on

50. Failing to express your sincere interest in the job

Interview Tips for the Career Changer

Prepare to answer the inevitable first and make-or-break question, "Why did you decide to change careers and pursue a career in the veterinary care field?"

- Write out the answer to why you are changing careers, and practice it many times so that you feel confident and comfortable answering it a considerable amount of time prior to interviewing. Many times there is considerable emotion surrounding this change, and it's best to have this resolved prior to interviewing.

- Describe in a *positive* way why you decided to change careers. Keep it simple and positive, even if there wasn't a particularly positive ending to your previous career.

- People make decisions for a variety of reasons. Relinquish any baggage from your past work life. It's okay to briefly acknowledge that your past circumstances were less than perfect, but keep it brief and simple.

- Show how the skills that you honed in your former career can transfer to the veterinary field. You will need to spend some time in outlining those skills and describing, using the STAR technique, how you can transfer those skills. You will most likely have your duties from your former jobs listed on a past resume.

- You do not need to have prior experience in the veterinary field to get a job in this field when you can describe your transferable skills as well as what you learned through you education and personal experience with animals.

- It is always preferable to have some volunteer experience with animals if possible, but it is not a requirement.

- Emphasize any past work experience dealing with the public. Employers in the veterinary field look for your ability to deal with clients as well as animals. Teaching of any kind is also looked upon as a positive, as well as problem solving.

- Describe how you learned a skill in the past when you had no prior experience to demonstrate that you have the ability to learn new procedures and techniques. You can also describe how many of the skills you have learned through your schooling were brand new, and describe how you have learned them through practice.

- Assure your interviewer that you have given a great deal of thoughtful consideration about venturing into this new career and convince them that this is what you truly want to do in your work life.

Dressing for the Interview in the Veterinary Field!

YES:

- Khakis, Docker-style or dark-colored dress pants (or skirt)
- Wrinkle-free buttoned shirt or golf shirt
- Clothes that fit properly
- Clean, closed-toed shoes
- Only one ring on each hand (other than engagement and wedding ring sets)
- Clean, neat hair, styled out of your eyes (If your hair is below your shoulders, it should be tied back or up neatly.)
- Clean, trimmed fingernails, natural or light-colored nail polish only
- Small earrings (studs) or very small loops only (if you normally wear earrings)
- Leggings only if the top is long enough to cover your backside
- *Specifically for men:* Wear an undershirt if you are wearing a buttoned shirt or light-colored golf shirt
- Wear a belt if your pants have belt hooks, and your shirt should be tucked in
- Shave the day of the interview, if you do not have a beard
- If you have a beard or mustache, have it neatly trimmed

NO:

- Blue jeans or white slacks
- Leather skirts, pants, blazers, or outdoor-type jackets
- Low-cut blouses or tops
- Sleeveless blouses
- Clothes that are too large or too small or tight
- Undergarments that show when wearing below-the-waist pants
- Dark undergarments that can be seen through light shirts or pants
- Wrinkled shirts or tops or those with sparkles or that shine
- T-shirts with short or long sleeves

- Low-cut pants where you can see skin when you sit down

- Bracelets or dangling earrings

- Facial piercings, especially tongue and nose rings

- Visible tattoos (cover them with clothing for the interview)

- Necklaces showing (you can tuck them into your shirt for the interview)

- Open-toed shoes, sandals, shoes with very high heels, or flip flops

- Multiple shades of hair color or unnatural-colored hair (depending on the city you are interviewing in)

- Knee socks with a skirt or dress

- Scrubs

- Perfume or cologne

*Turn off your cell phone, do not chew gum, and do not hold a
pen or pencil in your hand while interviewing.*

Your Job Interview!

THE DAY BEFORE THE INTERVIEW

- Know the name of the facility, the address, directions, and the approximate amount of time it will take you to get there.

- Make sure you know the time of the interview.

- Learn the name of the person who will be interviewing you.

- Make sure your interview clothes are clean, wrinkle free, and ready to go. (Try the outfit on several days prior to the interview.)

- Print out several copies of your resume, reference page, a list of questions to ask, and/or your portfolio.

- Get a blank thank-you card with a stamp on it.

- If you are driving your car, be sure to have plenty of gas, and make sure your car is clean. (Your interview begins when you drive into the parking lot!)

THE DAY OF THE INTERVIEW

- Give yourself plenty of time to prepare for the interview.

- Shower, brush your hair and teeth, use mouthwash and deodorant, and use eye drops if your eyes are red.

- Dress in your interview clothes.

- Go over your interview questions and answers.

- Take your portfolio or several copies of your resume and reference page, the name of facility, address, and directions, and the name of the person who will be interviewing you.

- Remember to take along your smile and confidence.

WHEN YOU ARRIVE FOR THE INTERVIEW

- If you are more than fifteen minutes early for your assigned interview time, stay in your car and review your questions. Be sure to turn off your phone at this time.

- When you go into the building, greet the person at the front desk with a smile, say your first and last name, and tell them that you have an _____(time) interview with _____ (name of interviewer). *You may need to wait until the person at the desk is not attending to customers.*

- You will either be directed or escorted to where you are to interview or be greeted by the interviewer in the waiting area

- You may be directed to sit and wait in the waiting area. If this is the case, be sure to go over your interview questions once again or to observe the activities and how the facility is operating.

- Do not take your phone out at this time. (Remember, you are being evaluated as soon as you get to the facility. Be sure to be upbeat and polite to the front desk person, but do not engage in a personal conversation with that person or the customers or the other staff members who may be in the area.)

WHEN GREETING YOUR INTERVIEWER

- Make eye contact, smile, and give a firm handshake. This will make an immediate statement about you.

- Be sure to get excited, not nervous, about the opportunity to interview for a job that you love!

- Remember that there is a job for everyone. This may or may not be the right fit, but you need to give it your best effort. Approach each interview with the mind-set that this is the job that you trained for and the job that you've wanted all of your life!

- A firm one-shake handshake, while looking into the eyes of the interviewer with a smile, will show confidence.

- A weak handshake using a wiggly wrist or a grasp of just the fingers does not show confidence and works against you from the start. Shaking several times is not necessary, and a very hard (possibly painful) grasp is not recommended.

- Remain standing until the interviewer suggests you take a seat. If the interviewer sits, then you can sit.

A FEW ACTIONS TO AVOID ON AN INTERVIEW

There are some bad habits that have been observed by interviewers:

- Leg bouncing
- Swiveling in chair
- Clicking a pen
- Twirling your hair around your fingers
- Putting your arms and/or elbows on the desk in front of you
- Swinging your leg when it is crossed
- Slouching

Have a trusted friend let you know if you tend to do these things when you are nervous.

STAGES OF THE INTERVIEW

- *First is the introductory stage of the interview.* There is generally a bit of small talk or breaking the ice banter in the first minute or two of an interview. (For example, did you have any trouble finding us? How was the traffic today on the way here? Do *not* complain about anything, even if you had to drive around for an hour before finding the facility or the traffic was backed for a mile due to an accident! Do not mention this. You can say that you didn't mind the drive, or you are used to traffic.)

- Next is the *information stage,* where the interviewer will most likely talk to you about the facility and possibly the staff and the services they provide. Many interviewers will ask *you* what you know about the facility before they go into detail (this is where your research comes in). You can impress them with what you know about them.

- *The getting to know you stage* comes next through questions about your interests, education, and job experience or simply by talking with you in general terms. (This is the stage where you need to be most alert and be sure you listen carefully and only answer the question that is asked. Inexperienced candidates sometimes ramble and give too much information, and others say too little, with one- or two-word answers or do not actually answer what is asked.) If you use the STAR format for answering all questions, you will be a star!

- *The closing stage* gives you a great opportunity to shine. Usually you will be asked if you have any questions. Use your prepared questions, and ask a minimum of two questions. If something the interviewer said needs clarification, this is the time to ask that also. What if the interviewer answered all you prepared questions? This is the time that you acknowledge what specific questions you were going to ask and let them know that they answered them, giving back to them their specific answer, indicating that you understood. Last, tell them that you are very interested in the position and when will they be making a hiring decision. Never leave an interview without some sort of timeline as to when you will be hearing from them. If they do not give you a specific date, ask if you can call them in a week to inquire about the progress of the hiring process.

THE TELEPHONE INTERVIEW

Regardless of the position you are applying for, employers in a service industry (such as veterinarians) want to check out your telephone skills.

Here are some things that employers listen for:

- If they get voice mail, is the message appropriate and friendly?
- Did the candidate turn his or her TV or music off or down when they called?
- Is he or she obviously eating, chewing gum, or smoking?
- Does he or she listen and answer the questions accordingly?
- How is the candidate's grammar, diction, and voice tone?

- Can you understand each other? This includes language, accent, volume, or tongue rings!

- Be sure to schedule a telephone interview.

- If an employer calls, do not agree if he or she says, "Let's do it right now, since I have you on the phone!"

SCHEDULED TELEPHONE INTERVIEW

A scheduled phone interview is an in-depth prescreen before the on-site interview. In some cases for externships, it is the actual interview and applicants are hired solely on the basis of the phone interview. Scheduled interviews can last anywhere from fifteen minutes to one hour.

HOW TO PREPARE

- Choose a place to conduct the phone interview without distractions. (If you have roommates or family members around, you may want to give them notice.)

- When you are using a cell phone, make sure you can get a signal in the chosen location.

- Check that your cell phone's battery is charged.

- Turn off call waiting.

- Keep your resume, portfolio, and job description (if you have one) in clear view. (Possibly tape it to your desk or a wall.)

- Make a short list of accomplishments or experiences you think the employer should know about you that makes the connection between your skills and the position.

- Have a pen and paper ready to take notes on questions and answers immediately after the phone interview.

- Practice with a trusted person who can give you honest feedback.

DURING THE TELEPHONE INTERVIEW

- Get dressed and cleaned up for the phone interview. Feeling like a professional will help you convey confidence.

- Your posture will affect how you sound. Sit up or stand while the interview is happening.

- Smiling can affect how you come across.

- You shouldn't have any food, drink, or gum, smoke, or wear a tongue ring during the interview.

- Speak clearly and enunciate.

- Always use the interviewer's title and last name.

- If you are having difficulty hearing the recruiter, let him or her know.
- Show that you are enthusiastic about the organization and the position.
- Build rapport with the interviewer. Be yourself, but always remain professional.
- Follow the interviewer's cues, and don't ramble to fill silences.
- Show that you are interested in the position by your voice and word choices.

ANTICIPATE THE INTERVIEW

- Research the facility.
- Review potential interview questions, and come up with possible answers using examples.
- Prepare questions to ask the interviewer.
- *Always* ask questions.

SUCCESSFUL PHONE INTERVIEW—SUMMARY

- Demonstrate a connection between your skills and the position.
- Answers questions thoughtfully, demonstrating you have done your research and are prepared.
- Show that you are articulate and conduct yourself professionally.
- Develop rapport with the recruiter, and demonstrate sincere interest in the position.
- You need to have your resume and portfolio in front of you, as well as a paper and pen to jot down notes while you are participating in a telephone interview.
- Arrange to be in a quiet place where there will be no interruptions or noise.

When to Start Your Job Search

You are in the throes of completing your externship, and you will be graduating when it's completed. You have a couple of more weeks to go. It looks like there a couple of technicians and assistants who don't seem to be very busy. There is talk that someone might be laid off work. It doesn't look like there is a job for you after your externship.

What do you do?

1. Ask your externship supervisor how you go about applying for a vet tech job at their facility. You will most likely be told one of the following.

    a. You will be told how their system works with externs applying by submitting your resume and/or filling out an application, or if they have other procedures in place. You may or may not need to interview for a position, since you completed your externship there, but in other cases, you will be interviewed along with other applicants.

    b. You will be told that there are no openings at this time, but you can apply for future openings.

    c. You will be told that there are not openings and no openings are anticipated in the near future. Therefore, you should apply elsewhere.

2. If you are told there are no anticipated openings, this is the time that you start your job search. This way you can get a jump on the students who are waiting until they are told that there are no openings, most likely the final day of their externship. If you feel that your externship was successful and you have been getting positive feedback, ask for a brief letter of recommendation, on the facility's letterhead, signed by your supervisor, veterinarian, or whomever can write about your experience as an extern there.

3. Create a list of facilities in the areas you have decided that you could travel to in order to work there daily. Include the name of the facility, address, email, fax, website, contact person, and brief description of what type of practice or research facility for each.

4. If your school offers a career services for graduates, contact them *as soon as you know* that you *will not be working at your externship site* upon completing you externship. Send them your updated resume (which includes your graduation date and your externship), along with your list of places you'd like to work. Ask if they know of any job openings in your area, and state the areas where you are able travel to work. If there are openings, look up those places and write a brief cover letter to those who have openings to a specific person. Contact your career services representative once a week to give them updates, or retrieve any updates on other openings.

5. If you get called for an interview from one of the facilities your career services representative sent your resume to, be sure to let them know that you have an interview scheduled. If you are offered a second interview, and then a job, let the career services representative know that also.

Dos and Don'ts for Effective Job Hunting in the Veterinary Field

There are common misconceptions concerning the most
effective ways to job search in the *veterinary field*

Do research on <u>each</u> facility to which you will be applying. Select a few interesting facts from your research and put it in your cover letter, to show that you are a good fit for their facility. Veterinary facilities most often rely on local tech schools to supply them with resumes or ask other employees if they can recommend someone. At times, there is a bonus offered for employees who find job candidates who get hired.

Do make a list of all of the veterinary practices in your area, adding the name of the practice manager, office manager, or hospital manager, if listed. If none of these are listed, select the veterinarian who is the owner. If that is not listed, and there are many doctors on the website, select the first one. Addressing a cover letter "To Whom This May Concern" shows you did not take the time to research the facility.

Do research all on the list and mention something about the practice in your cover letter. Write a paragraph that is unique to each practice and mention why you would like to work there. Writing an individual cover letter for each place that you apply only involves changing one paragraph. The rest of the letter can remain the same. Be very careful to keep them organized so you send the correct letter to the correct practice!

Do send a brief cover letter along with your resume when applying for jobs.

Do make sure you have a teacher, trusted family member, or friend review your cover letter for errors.

Do look online to see which clinics are hiring veterinarians. If you are still in school and have several months remaining to complete your degree, keep notes of those places that are hiring veterinarians, and apply when you are nearing your graduation to those places. If they are adding a veterinarian to their staff, they often need addition veterinary support staff.

Don't only apply to jobs listed online. (There is an extensive hidden job market in the veterinary field.)

Don't skip applying to jobs that say hiring those with experience and/or licensed preferred, if you have just graduated from a school with a certificate or degree. The employer often puts on the advertisement for employees what they ideally would like to hire, but if they do not get resumes from individuals with those qualifications, then they will go to the next best person. *It could be you!* If you are not yet licensed but are eligible to become licensed through your education, add that to your resume or cover letter.

Don't call veterinary clinics and ask if they have job openings. Usually clinics are busy, and the person answering the phone is juggling many tasks and also may not be in the loop about the hiring process. The easiest way to get someone off of the telephone is simply to say, "No, we are not hiring," which may not be the case at all. It is discouraging when you call several places and feel that there are no job openings! Skip that step and email, fax, or stop in and drop off your cover letter and resume. This is much more effective.

Don't send your reference page along with your resume unless you are specifically asked to do so. Bring it along to the interview, but do not offer it unless asked.

Don't attend job fairs. Sometimes job fairs can be fun, but with the internet to research facilities, there really isn't a reason to go from one booth to another and talk to someone while you both are standing with many other activities going on around you.

A few words about Facebook, hair color, and piercings when it comes to your job search.

FACEBOOK

There are a great many employers who make a practice of checking a candidate's Facebook page before deciding to call them in for an interview. Remember, when you are working in the veterinary field, you represent the entire clinic, hospital, research facility, or wherever you may be working. There have been students who lost their opportunity to be hired by their externship site due to what they posted on their Facebook page about concerns they had about certain clinic procedures they did not happen to agree with. Another graduate was not granted an interview due to the fact that she had dozens of pictures of herself on her Facebook page. There were no problem pictures, but the interviewer felt that this person was too much about herself and would not be a team player in a clinic setting. It is very simple. Do not put off potential employers by posting questionable content. Be sure that your privacy settings don't broadcast your updates to those outside of your friends list. If you do add potential employers and colleagues, use groups to keep professional contacts separate from family and friends or mark your posts so they will only be visible for close friends and family.

PIERCINGS AND HAIR COLOR (MAY VARY IN DIFFERENT AREAS)

The issue is *not* having those things. The issue is displaying them!

- Consider that green hair (or whatever unnatural hair color or multiple hair colors), tattoos, and various piercings are not going to *help* you get a job, unless it's in an artsy industry. However, having those things *can hurt you*.

- Why set yourself up to possibly be hurt by something in your job search, especially when you are just starting out in a new career?

- Why risk alienating people? There are other qualified people who *don't* have those distracting adornments who will be more attractive candidates.

- There is the issue of self-expression. Remember, this is *work*. Work is not about *you* or your expression of yourself. No one cares.

- Do what needs to be done at work. Express yourself on your own time.

IN CONCLUSION

Finding a job in the veterinary care field or any field is very systematic. It's not just a matter of luck or who you or your parents or your friends happen to know. Luck is being prepared to take advantage of opportunities that are presented to you. If you prepare the tools you need to be a successful job searcher that are outlined in this book, you will make your own luck!

The internet has obviously changed how resumes and applications are being sent to employers, although you still need to have the information presented in a concise, orderly manner. That hasn't changed. Styles have changed, and what you wear on an interview has changed over the years. What has not changed is dressing neatly and modestly. Referrals from a previous employer still mean a great deal to a prospective employer. Developing a career portfolio and continuing to add to it as your career progresses is a stress-free way of being prepared for future opportunities when they arise. Keep your portfolio current, by first updating your resume as soon as your accept a new job and keeping track of your accomplishments at work. This will be very helpful when it comes to your yearly evaluation. A current portfolio can be a factor in your receiving a raise or being accepted into a future educational program.

Over the years hiring managers in the veterinary field are constantly adding and replacing veterinary care support staff due to the tremendous growth in the industry. They have a demanding and very busy job. Be patient during the hiring process. While waiting for a call after an interview, continue to send your resume to other facilities.

Remember, all employers need good, qualified workers and desperately *want to hire you*. Your job in the interview is to make it *easy* for them to make that happen by following what is outlined in this book.

Best of everything and much success in pursuing the career that you love!

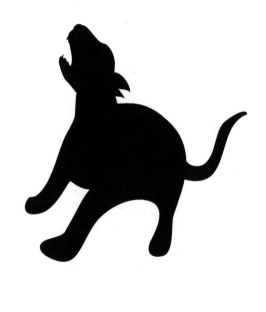

About the Author

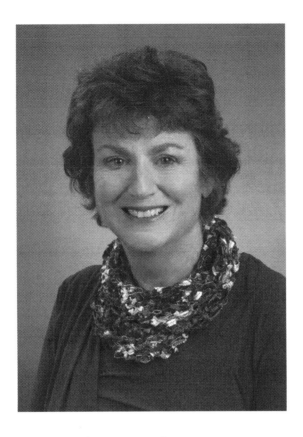

Patricia M. Lee, MA (Pat), has over thirty years of experience as a career counselor in a variety of educational settings and takes great pride in offering individuals a step-by-step approach to finding a job of their dreams. Pat earned a bachelor's degree in psychology and a master's degree in counseling and student services. For over a decade, she has served as the director of career placement for Vet Tech Institute in Pittsburgh, where Pat has successfully assisted students find careers in the veterinary care field. As an avid animal lover, she has rescued almost every pet she has owned. Mrs. Lee resides in Washington, Pennsylvania, with her husband, two pit bull/boxer rescue dogs, a miniature donkey, and a registered paint mare that she rides every chance she gets.

Printed in the United States
By Bookmasters